# Home Remedies That Work

Safer, Cheaper Herbal & Natural Remedies
for Healthy Living

by

*Jim Long*

Copyright© 2012, Jim Long

All rights reserved. No portion of this book may be reproduced without written permission from the author, except for review; nor may any part of this book be reproduced, stored in a retrieval system, or transmitted in any form or by any means, including electronic, mechanical, photocopying, internet or other, without written permission from the author.

Published by

Long Creek Herbs
P.O. Box 127
Blue Eye, MO 65611

Printed in the United States by Multi-Printing, Forsyth, Missouri

ISBN 978-1-889791-09-8

# HOME REMEDIES THAT WORK

*Safer, Cheaper, Natural Alternatives for Healthy Living*

This information is solely for informational purposes. It is not intended to provide medical advice. Always consult a reliable reference before using any plant or herb and be certain of the correct identification. Exercise all precautionary measures while following instructions on home remedies in this book; avoid using any plants or products if you are allergic to them. Always consult a qualified medical person for questions about any disease or ailment.

These are folk remedies I've collected over the years from various sources. Some are my own formulas I've used myself, others were recommended by friends or reliable sources. Always use caution with any folk remedy and consult a physician or qualified health provider for any questionable or serious illness.

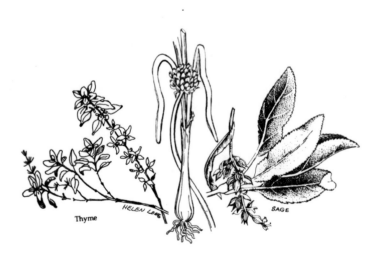

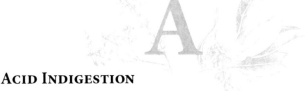

## Acid Indigestion

The best remedy is Mint tea. Anti-acid tablets such as Rolaids® contain calcium carbonate (chalk) and peppermint oil, among other ingredients. Dried or fresh mint tea helps soothe an upset stomach. Fennel tea or chewing fennel seeds, also works.

## Acid Reflux

Frequent acid reflux is known as gastroesophageal reflux disease, or GERD. Acid in the stomach is natural and necessary for digestion and prevents germs from getting into the lungs; nightly heartburn, coughing, nausea and trouble swallowing might be symptoms of GERD. Avoiding fatty foods, as well as onions, tomatoes and chocolate may be helpful. Consult a doctor if you have symptoms worse than ordinary heartburn.

**Apple cider vinegar and fresh Ginger** is a simple and cheap remedy. Mix 1/2 cup apple cider vinegar and 1 teaspoon fresh ginger in a blender then strain. Drink a tablespoonful. Most people feel relief in 2-3 minutes.

According to Anahad O'Connor, writing in *The New York Times*, chewing one or two pieces of **gum** can relieve ordinary heartburn. "Chewing on a piece of gum helps force fluids back into the stomach and flood the esophagus with alkaline saliva, neutralizing acids that cause the characteristic burning sensations," he wrote.

For some people, **raising the head of the bed** higher than the foot is also helpful. (Dr. Zorba Paster of *Zorba Paster on Your Health*, a popular radio show on Public Radio (wpr.org/zorba), recommends stopping chewing gum because Dr. Zorba says you are taking air into your stomach when you chew gum which can contribute to acid reflux). It's conflicting advice, meaning one works for some people, while the opposite may be helpful for others.

***Slippery Elm*** is often effective for acid reflux, according to Liz Lipski, PhD, and author of *Digestive Wellness*. Slippery elm coats the throat and stomach and can relieve inflammation in the intestines. Slippery elm tablets are available in most whole foods stores or the supplement aisle of your pharmacy.

## Arthritis

An old folk remedy for arthritis was ***Cayenne Pepper***, rubbed on the affected area. A story reported in the *American Journal of Clinical Nutrition*, 2009, says that capsaicin ointments and creams are beneficial for easing muscle aches, pain and arthritis. Capsaicin is the oil of cayenne pepper. - use an over-the-counter capsaicin cream.

**Arthritis Poultice** - The late Jerry Stamps, an apothecary-pharmacist, recommend this: Mix 6 tablespoons Mullein leaves *(Verbascum thapsus)*, 9 tablespoons Slippery Elm bark *(Ulmus rubra)*, 3 tablespoons Lobelia *(Lobelia siphilitica)* and 1 tablespoon Cayenne Pepper. Store in air-tight container. **To use**: Take out 2 tablespoons of the mixture and add just enough boiling water to make a paste. Spread on a cloth and apply to the affected area. Cover with another warm cloth and leave for 20-30 minutes. Label the mixture, EXTERNAL USE ONLY, as it isn't safe to use internally.

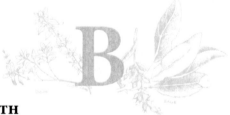

## Bad Breath

Drinking a hot cup of ***unsweetened black tea*** helps. This remedy is especially useful if the bad breath is caused by dry mouth or "morning" breath.

Bad breath is sometimes caused by poor digestion rather than a problem in the mouth. Eating ***yogurt*** on a regular basis can help. Rinsing your mouth with the juice of half a ***fresh lemon*** in lukewarm water is also helpful.

Persistent bad breath may be an indication of something else going on in the body. One Amish remedy claimed that a yeast infection in the lining of the stomach could be a cause and *removing bread, milk, fruit juice and sugars* from the diet can make a big difference. Many people report amazing results by leaving these foods out of their daily diets.

Chewing fresh *Parsley* is an excellent breath freshener due to its odor-absorbing chlorophyll and it's been an old stand-by since ancient Roman times. Chewing a *coffee bean* is also effective. In a pinch, lick *stainless steel* to remove offensive breath!

## Bed Bugs

**Bed Bugs** die when sprayed with a mixture of 1 part Dawn (original) Dish Soap with 5 parts water.

## Bed Sores, early stages

Bed sores are a common occurrence for anyone hospitalized for long periods, especially the elderly. Here's a simple recipe that sounds strange, but is said to actually help heal and bring relief. (Bed sores should be seen by a medical person).

*1/8 cup powdered sugar* combined with enough Barbasol brand shave cream to make a paste. Apply liberally several times daily. Gently wash area before applying. For whatever reason, Barbasol seems to work best.

*Powdered sugar with enough honey* to make a paste, apply it twice daily, gently washing the wound before each application. *Vitamin E Oil*, applied to the area can also be helpful.

## Bee Sting

*Meat tenderizer* applied to the sting area stops the hurt in seconds. A piece of *banana peel*, applied white side on the skin, held in place with tape is also effective.

## Bitten Tongue

It's painful when you accidentally bite your tongue or burn it on too-hot food. Try a *cough lozenge* that contains benzocaine to lessen the pain.

Sucking on a cool, *wet black tea bag* is also effective. The tannin released from the tea bag has a pain-relieving effect and slows bleeding, too. *Plain honey* held in the mouth also works.

## Bleeding

*Yarrow* - This amazing blood-stopping herb has been used since the time of the ancient Greeks on battlefield wounds. Crush fresh leaves and apply as a poultice or use the dried leaves or flowers, powdered, and applied directly to the wound.

*Note:* Yarrow stops bleeding so fast it can trap debris in the wound so be sure to clean the wound thoroughly. *Turmeric* - Apply the dried powder or fresh root directly to stop bleeding.

## Blood Pressure

*Bananas!* - They're extremely high in potassium yet low in salt, making them perfect to help lower blood pressure. So much so, the US Food and Drug Administration allows the banana industry to make official claims for the fruit's ability to reduce the risk of blood pressure and stroke. (Lots of things contribute to blood pressure, always consult a physician).

## Body Odor

Diet has a lot to do with body odor. A diet high in beef, fast foods or overly-processed foods, increases body odor significantly. Eating more *spinach, collard greens, brussels sprouts, Parsley, cucumbers, string beans, asparagus or endive* can help. Adding *active culture yogurt* to the diet on a daily basis, is also helpful.

A folk remedy from Vietnam - Buy a "hand" (we think of it as the root) of *fresh Ginger*. Cut the ginger into chunks and put it in a food processor. Add 3 cups of water and pulverize the ginger. Pour through a sieve and let drain for 30 minutes. After showering, apply some of the liquid under the armpits. Save remaining ginger water in the refrigerator and use after every shower. **Raw turnip juice** will also work.

Eating 1 or 2 **bananas** daily helps with body odor, as does eating a few tablespoons of **active culture yogurt**.

## Boils

Boils are caused by bacterial infection, especially staphylococcus bacteria, and usually begin in a hair follicle. If you have skin boils, don't "pop" them as it might result in more serious infection. Instead, soak area in a warm bath 3 times a day and apply a warm Parsley Poultice, twice daily. Parsley Poultice - Mash fresh Parsley with the bottom of a spoon so that you have about 4 tablespoons of pulp. Wrap that in a damp washcloth, warm it in a microwave for 30 seconds and apply, holding it in place for 15 minutes.

*Cumin* - Mix 1 teaspoon ground Cumin with enough hot water to make a paste. Apply and leave in place for 15 minutes. Repeat 3 - 4 times daily.

*Cabbage Leaf* - Heat an outer leaf from a head of cabbage in the microwave and apply it while still warm to the area. Repeat several times daily.

*Onion* - Onions were so important as a wound remedy during the Civil War that every doctor kept them available. Onions have antibiotic properties that are useful with boils. Slice an onion in half and roast it in the oven for about 10 minutes (375 degrees F). After cooling, hold it in a washcloth and apply the cut side directly on the boil. Repeat 2 - 3 times each day.

## Brittle Nails

**Horsetail tea** *(Equisetum arvense)* is a natural home remedy that is said to be highly effective in strengthening brittle nails. Chris Kilham teaches ethnobotany at the University of Massachusetts Amherst, where he is the "Explorer In Residence," and is an adviser to herbal, cosmetic and pharmaceutical companies. "This (horsetail) is one of the simplest remedies I know, and works within just a couple of weeks," he said. "Drink two or more cups daily (horsetail tea) - you find that it does make a significant difference in both the appearance and strength of nails....One side benefit is your hair will also become more healthy," he said. Horsetail is naturally high in silica which is necessary for healthy nails, skin and hair.

*Note:* Those who are pregnant or have kidney problems should avoid using this and it's not intended for long term use.

***To make horsetail tea:*** Pour 1 cup boiling water over 2 teaspoons dry horsetail herb. Cover cup and let steep for 5 minutes. Stain out and discard horsetail and drink, sweetened or unsweetened. Two cups a day is the generally recommended amount.

***Fingernail Hardener*** - Combine 3 tablespoons water, 1 tablespoon glycerin with 1 teaspoon powdered alum. Store in airtight container until ready to use. Before bedtime, coat your nails with the mixture with a small brush. Let dry overnight. Remove from nails the following morning with rubbing alcohol and use a moisturizing hand lotion.

## BRUISES

***Banana Peel*** - Apply a banana peel, white side toward the flesh, held in place with a piece of tape, overnight.

## BURNS

Immediately after a burn, hold the area under running ***cool, but not ice cold, water*** to keep it from getting worse. Serious burns, of course, should be treated by a physician, but first-degree burns, those in which the skin isn't broken, like sunburn, can easily be treated at home. ***Aloe vera*** is an effective treatment. Apply it liberally over the burn.

*Note:* any kind of burn regardless of severity, heals faster if you drink plenty of ***water*** and restrict sodium intake. Add a multivitamin to your diet, as well, to aid in healing. If aloe vera isn't available, use ***toothpaste***. Also, ***Soy Sauce*** applied immediately is very helpful, according to military battlefield medics.

## BURNT TONGUE

Half a spoonful of ***plain sugar*** brings relief. ***Plain honey*** is also helpful.

## Burn from Eating Hot Pepper

Accidentally eat a too-hot pepper? *Sour cream, yogurt, milk, ice cream* or a half teaspoon of *sugar or honey*, will soothe the sting. Drinking water is the worst thing to do.

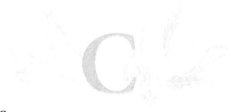

## Canker Sores

A simple treatment is to hold a pinch of *instant coffee crystals* on the sore spot. It's also helpful to rinse the mouth with *warm water and baking soda* several times a day. Many people report reduced incidence of canker sores after eating 2 - 4 tablespoons of *active culture yogurt* a day. A pinch of Turmeric applied to the area is also helpful.

## Chigger Bite

Bruise a leaf of *Plantain (Plantago major* or *P. lanceolata)* and hold it on the bite. The itching should disappear in seconds. If that isn't available, put a dab of *Preparation H* on the bite. The inside of a *banana peel* applied to bite also brings fast relief.

## Constipation

*Prune juice* is one of the easiest and safest short-term remedies. Constipation is often caused by poor diet without fresh fruits, vegetables and grains.

A longer-term remedy is a *high-fiber diet* combined with about 1/3 cup of *active culture yogurt* daily. High-fiber foods such as whole-grain bread, beans, broccoli, peas, cauliflower and apples help maintain gastrointestinal health and ward off constipation. High-fiber diets can often cause unwanted gas, which is why the yogurt is important.

Eat a *banana* before bedtime - Bananas are high in fiber and help ease constipation.

## Coughing

***Horehound Cough Drops*** - This old time formula still works. Modern day horehound cough drops seldom contain any horehound, but are "flavored" with artificial flavoring which does nothing to stop coughing or a sore throat. You can make your own:

### *Horehound Cough Drops*

> 8 cups water
> 1/2 cup dried horehound leaves or leaves & flowering tops
> 4 cups sugar
> 1 1/4 cups dark cane syrup
> 1 tablespoon butter
> 1 teaspoon cream of tartar

*Also have ready:*

> Candy thermometer
> 
> Cookie sheet that has sides, or any shallow pan the size of a cookie sheet, with sides
> 
> 1 tablespoon extra butter
> 1/8 cup extra sugar

Butter the cookie sheet with the extra tablespoon of butter and set aside.

Bring the 8 cups of water to a boil and immediately remove pan from heat. Add the horehound herb, cover pan with a lid and let the liquid cool for 20 minutes. Strain through a tea strainer or cheesecloth and discard the herb.

To the liquid, add the remaining ingredients. Cook over medium-high heat until the liquid reaches the hard-crack stage (300 degrees F. on a candy thermometer). Remove from heat and immediately pour it into the buttered cookie pan.

As the candy begins to cool - this takes less than a minute - quickly score the candy with a knife dipped in water. Score quickly into bite-sized "drops" or "lozenges," about 1/2 inch by 1 inch - cough drop size. The candy will harden fast. In about 5 minutes the candy can be broken along the scored lines. As soon as you've broken the cough drops apart, toss them in the extra sugar. This prevents them from sticking together. Leave in the air to dry for about an hour then store in an air-tight container.

*Ginger tea with honey*. Research suggests that compounds in ginger are as effective as most over the counter cough remedies. *Thyme tea* is also an excellent cough remedy. The herb, Thyme *(Thymus sp.)* has been used for centuries as a cough suppressant. Sweeten with honey if desired.

## COUGHING, DRY

This remedy has been used in India for centuries. Mix 1 tablespoon of **Turmeric powder** with about 1 teaspoon **honey**. Put about a fourth teaspoonful in the mouth and suck on it slowly so it coats the throat.

## COUGHING WITH A COLD AND CONGESTION

*Hot tea with honey* is soothing to the throat and there is some clinical evidence to support its use, according to Mark Yoder, MD, who is a Pulmonary Care specialist at Rush University Medical Center in Chicago. It's also important to drink plenty of fluids, like water or tea but avoid soft drinks which often make phlegm worse.

Make a chest rub - Put 10 drops **Eucalyptus essential oil**, 10 **drops Spearmint essential oil** in a shot glass (2 oz.) of canola or corn oil. Massage on chest 2 or 3 times a day.

## COUGHING, NIGHTTIME

Apply **Vicks Vaporub**®, to the bottoms of the feet, then pull on socks to hold it on. Lots of people swear by this remedy!

## CRACKING HEEL

Cracking heel is actually a form of athlete's foot known as *tinea pedis*, the same fungus that causes jock itch. It's painful; often the skin cracks and bleeds on the heel and between the toes. No amount of lotions, grinding or filing away the rough edges will make it go away. A very simple formula that is guaranteed to work in about 2 weeks is **Herbal Nail Fungus Soak**, available from LongCreekHerbs.com. It's my own formula containing several antifungal herbs shown to be effective on a variety of fungal conditions.

## CUTS & SCRAPES

**Turmeric powder** is a blood-stopping remedy used in India for centuries. Simply sprinkle the dry turmeric powder on the wound. It is said to stop bleeding and start healing immediately. For tiny nicks like shaving or paper cuts, rub on a bit of **lip balm**. For slightly larger cuts, a good remedy in a pinch is **honey**. Honey contains antibacterial properties, helps prevent infection and speeds healing. **Honey combined with Turmeric** is even better.

An ancient Greek Remedy - **Yarrow** *(Achillea millefolium)* - Use dry or fresh, leaves and/or flowers. The herb was named in honor of Achillies, the Greek warrior in the Trojan War. Legend says his mother held him by the left heel when he was a baby, dunking him in the River Styx to make him impervious to wounds. His heel was the only part not protected. As an adult he was killed by an arrow in the heel. The folk tale was concocted to remind people how important yarrow was to ancient battlefield doctors. **To use:** Bruise a fresh leaf and apply it directly to a wound. Or, as was done by folk healers during the Civil War, use dried, powdered leaves or flowers and sprinkle on the bleeding wound.

*Note:* this herb works so quickly it can seal debris in the injury, so be sure to clean the wound first. Yarrow stops bleeding in seconds.

Canadian Wound Remedy - Place a **wet teabag** on a wound to stop bleeding.

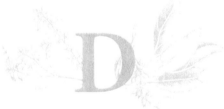

## DANDRUFF

Mix 2 cups plain **apple cider vinegar** with 1/2 cup warm water. Pour over just-washed hair, wrap hair in a towel and leave on for 5 minutes. Rinse. Repeat 3 times a week until dandruff is gone - usually in a couple of weeks or less.

For really bad dandruff or red patches in beard or mustache: Mix 1/4 cup **Shavegrass**, 2 tablespoons **Lemon Balm**, 2 tablespoons

*Lavender*, 1 tablespoon *Thyme* with 4 cups barely simmering apple cider vinegar. Let simmer for 2 minutes, remove from heat, cover with a lid and let cool overnight. Next day, strain and discard herbs, then add 2 cups water. For places on face or beard, apply several times daily with cotton ball or wash cloth. For hair, pour through, cover with a towel and leave on for 15 minutes. Don't rinse out.

## DEPRESSION

There are lots of reasons for depression but in a study from the University of Wisconsin, Madison, researchers found that pleasant smells can have a positive effect on easing depression. Put 2 drops of **Peppermint essential oil** along the back of your neck. Next, inhale about 10 deep breaths of the peppermint oil, placed under your nose. Of course, for serious depression, seek medical help or counseling.

It's also helpful to eat a ***banana***. Bananas contain tryptophan, a type of protein that the body converts into serotonin, long known to help you relax and improve mood. One-fourth cup of Lavender flowers tied in a cloth and placed under the pillow where you sleep is also helpful.

## DIARRHEA

***Burnt toast*** - Toast any kind of bread until it is seriously black, then break it in pieces and eat. (See also, charcoal, below).

***Green banana*** - Eat 2-4 green bananas a day to stop diarrhea.

***Charcoal Capsules*** - You'll find purified charcoal capsules in health food stores. Take 2-4 capsules after every bout of diarrhea, swallowing with a cup of water. It should clear up in about a day. If not, consult your doctor immediately.

***Blackberry Leaves*** - Pick two or three blackberry leaves. Tear leaves in pieces and pour 1/2 cup boiling water over and let steep for 5 minutes. Strain and drink. Blackberry leaves have been used for diarrhea for centuries.

***Apples*** - Peel and grate an apple onto a plate, spread it out then leave it until it has turned brown, about 30 minutes. Eat the grated apple and take a nap. This relieves the stomach gurgling and the nap helps you relax.

# Diaper Rash

*(See Rashes, and also Calendula Salve under Skin Problems)*

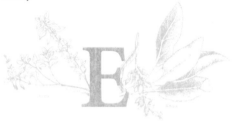

# Earache

Ear pain is often the sign of infection and should be treated by your doctor. In the meantime, try **warm oil**. Simple olive oil with a few drops of liquid garlic extract is a good choice. Warm the oil to just barely above normal body temperature, then lay your head on the side with your painful ear up and put a few drops of warm oil into the ear canal. Leave it for a few minutes, then turn your head and let drain.

Half-fill a clean handkerchief with **table salt**, tie it closed and microwave for about 30 seconds. Apply it while very warm to the painful ear for several minutes.

# Erectile Dysfunction

L-arginine, an amino acid found naturally in meat, fish and poultry is available as an oral supplement that some manufacturers sell as a "natural Viagra." Studies show 5 grams a day over a six week period to be effective.

# Eyes, Puffy

**Cucumber** - Apply a thin slice of cucumber to each closed eyelid. Leave on for 10 minutes and the eyes will feel better. A used, **wet tea bag**, placed over the closed eyelids, works, too; lie down and apply to closed eyelids, leave in place 10 minutes and the puffiness will disappear. **Preparation H,** works, too, just be careful to keep it out of your eyes.

## FLATULENCE, GAS

*Fennel tea* - Bring 2 cups of water to a boil. Add 1 tablespoon fennel seed and simmer for 2 minutes. Strain and drink. You can also chew and swallow a teaspoon of fennel seed, which is also good for indigestion.

*Peppermint tea* - If you've eaten a large meal, to help prevent embarrassing gas, drink a cup of hot peppermint tea and take a brisk walk. *Yogurt* is also helpful, especially if you have a high-fiber diet. Yogurt helps break down gas and aids digestion.

## FLEAS ON PETS OR PEOPLE

*Dawn (original) Dishwashing Liquid* is very effective. Use 1 teaspoon in the bathwater for a large dog, 1/2 teaspoon for a small dog. Wash, then rinse well, making sure none of the soap remains. Use conditioner to keep the pets' skin from drying out and don't use more often than once a month. For people, use the soap in a washcloth, then rinse well. This doesn't prevent fleas but it does kill those that come in contact with the soapy water.

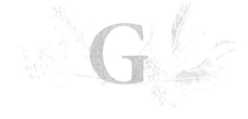

## GOUT

Mild gout can often be stopped by drinking sour *cherry juice*. One 6 ounce glass twice a day is often recommended. Use pure, sour cherry, or black cherry juice, available in whole foods stores. Pain of gout is brought on by build up of uric acid, which forms crystals, usually in the joints of the feet. Avoiding certain foods can keep gout from occurring: gravies, mushrooms, dry beans, red wine, spinach, sardines and organ meats can bring on a flare-up. Gout is a symptom of problems with the kidneys.

***Avoid beer and liquor*** if you are prone to gout. Alcohol raises the uric acid level in the blood and can bring on a flare-up. Alcohol can also cause you to be dehydrated, another gout trigger, so drink plenty of water to keep your system hydrated, which helps wash out uric acid. Sugary beverages containing fructose can also worsen gout flare-ups.

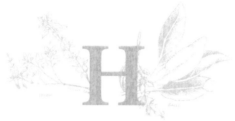

## Hair Conditioning

Several things help keep the hair looking healthy: ***Cool Whip*** rubbed into the hair and left for 15 minutes then rinsed out. ***Beer*** poured through the hair after shampooing. Leave in for 5 minutes and rinse. Repeat once a week, then switch to once a month. Just-brewed ***iced tea*** (not instant), also works.

***Chamomile tea***, brewed strong, helps lighten hair. Bring 6 cups of water to a boil, add 1 heaping cup of dried Chamomile flowers, stir and simmer for 2 minutes. Remove from heat, cover with a lid and let set overnight. The following day, strain and discard the herbs. To the liquid, add 2 teaspoons of lemon juice or distilled white vinegar. Keep refrigerated until ready to use. Slightly warm 2 cups of the solution and pour through just-washed hair. Leave on 5 minutes then rinse.

***Rosemary rinse*** for darker hair: Bring 6 cups of water to a boil. Add 1 cup of dried ***Rosemary Leaves***. Simmer for 2 minutes, remove pan from heat, cover with a lid over night. The following day, strain out and discard the herbs. Add 1 tablespoon of apple cider vinegar. Keep liquid refrigerated until ready to use. Slightly warm 2 cups of the liquid and pour through just-shampooed hair. Leave on 5 minutes then rinse.

## Hair, Split Ends, Damaged Hair

Two teaspoons **Horsetail** *(Equisetum arvense)* steeped in 1 cup boiling water for 5 minutes, strain and drink twice daily for about 2 weeks, and in addition, use any of the hair conditioning treatments, above. Those who are pregnant or have kidney problems should avoid drinking this tea. It's also not meant for long-term use.

## Hangover

The quickest remedy for a hangover is a ***banana milkshake***, sweetened with ***honey.*** Bananas calm the stomach and honey helps build up the blood sugar levels while the milk rehydrates the body.

## Heartburn

*Ginger tea* - Bring 2 cups of water to a boil. Add 1 tablespoon chopped fresh ginger and simmer for 5 minutes. Strain, sweeten with honey if desired. Take 1-2 tablespoons as needed. Candied ginger - Chew a piece of candied ginger several times daily for heartburn. Avoid candied ginger if diabetic, or use only small amounts due to the sugar.

Drink 1 tablespoon of apple ***cider vinegar.*** The effect is almost immediate. Add a tiny bit of honey if you choose. The vinegar will burn going down for a second or two, then you will find the heartburn is gone.

## Hemorrhoids

*A diet too low in fiber is often a cause of constipation and results in hemorrhoids. Fixing the diet is the best cure.*

## Hemorrhoids, External

***Cumin Seed Paste*** - Make a paste by mixing ground cumin seed with enough water to moisten and apply the paste to the painful piles. ***Baking Soda*** - If the hemorrhoids have an itchy feeling, try applying a baking soda and water paste.

***Liquid Blistex***, applied just as you would ***Preparation H***. Or a slice of ***tomato***, left if place for an hour. ***Vitamin E oil*** is also helpful.

## HEMORRHOIDS, INTERNAL
### BLEEDING FROM THE INSIDE

*Dry Figs* - Eating figs twice daily is effective. The small seeds in this fruit helps in bowel movement and avoids constipation. Soak 4 figs in water overnight and eat them the next morning together with the water. Prepare another 4 figs in the morning and keep those for the evening. Repeat twice daily for 3 to 4 weeks.

*Coriander seed tea* - This helps stop bleeding when passing stools. Soak 2 teaspoons Coriander seeds in a glass of hot water over night and drink it the next morning. Drink twice daily for 4 or 5 days.

## HERPES, GENITAL OR ORAL

*Lemon balm* *(Melissa officinalis)*. According to New York University Medical Center (med.nyu.edu), "Topical lemon balm is most popular today as a treatment for genital or oral herpes." Lemon balm cream can be used topically but making a strong decoction (tea) and using it as a mouthwash several times daily is also helpful (for oral herpes). Pour 2 cups boiling water over 1/4 cup dried lemon balm. Cover and let cool for an hour. Use as a mouthwash, keep extra in the refrigerator. Drinking a daily cup of **lemon balm tea** is also helpful.

## HICCUPS

*Dill tea*. A teaspoon of Dill seeds added to a cup of just-boiled water. Cover cup with a saucer for 5 minutes, then strain and drink.

Dr. Jonas Richel, writing in *The Indian Physician*, in 1828, recommended 3 drops of **Peppermint oil** on a sugar cube. That's still a good remedy for hiccups and heartburn. If peppermint oil isn't available, use 2 or 3 drops of **Mint extract** from the kitchen spice shelf.

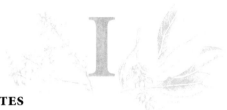

## INSECT BITES

*Banana peel*, apply white side next to the skin; or, sprinkle *Adolph's Meat Tenderizer* on affected area. *Preparation H* rubbed on the bite, or a *slice of tomato*, held in place for several minutes, also works.

*Plantain* (Plantago major), a common yard "weed" has been used since at least the 12th-century to help heal insect stings, bites, wounds and burns. Be sure of correct identity of the herb. Pick and bruise a leaf and hold it on the insect bite for a couple of minutes. Re-apply as necessary. An alternative method: Pour 2 cups boiling water over 1/2 cup of dried plantain, cover and let steep for 20 minutes. Strain and discard the herb. Dip a clean wash cloth in the liquid and apply it to the affected area, repeating as necessary.

## ITCHING EYES
(SEE ALSO PINKEYE)

Eyes that itch due to fatigue from reading, watching television or sitting in front of the computer can be helped by lightly *washing* the area around the eyes with mild soap and water, then applying a warm, fairly hot washcloth over the eyes and leaving in place for 2 minutes. Repeat 2 or 3 times during the day and take breaks to avoid continually straining your eyes.

## IRRITABLE BOWEL SYNDROME - CHRONIC DIARRHEA

*Coconut* is helpful. Some people report eating 2 *coconut macaroon cookies* daily controls chronic diarrhea. Drinking coconut water or milk is also known to be helpful.

Note: Be sure to consult with your doctor if you have chronic diarrhea to determine the cause.

*Diet* - cutting back on sugar, caffeine, citrus, spicy foods or wheat products, is helpful for some people. Researchers at Mayo Clinic say that adding more fiber to the diet is often helpful (and adding 2-3 tablespoons of *active culture yogurt* daily helps with gas that may result). They also recommend eating smaller meals and drinking plenty of *water* each day.

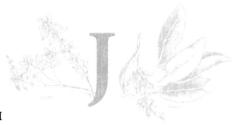

## Jock Itch

Jock itch is a fungal infection known as *tinea cruris*. An effective **Jock Itch Remedy** - Combine these dry herbs: 1/2 cup Shavegrass *(Equisetum arvense)*, 1/4 cup Plantain *(Plantago major)*, 2 tablespoons Thyme, 2 tablespoons Lavender flowers and 1 tablespoon Thyme with 5 cups apple cider vinegar, in a non-corrosive pan *(that means not aluminum nor cast iron)*. Bring vinegar to boiling, remove from heat, cover pan with a lid and let cool over night. Strain and discard herbs. **To use:** Apply to groin area with wash cloth, leaving in place for 5 minutes. Apply twice daily and the jock itch will be gone in about 2 weeks. Keep area dry between times, using the Absorbent Powder (listed under, *Rashes, Adult)*.

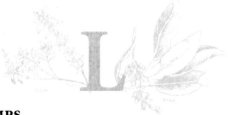

## Leg Cramps

Heat 1 cup *apple cider vinegar* to nearly boiling and remove from heat. Into the hot liquid add 1 tablespoon thinly sliced or diced *fresh Ginger root*. Let cool overnight. Strain and drink 1 to 2 tablespoons when leg cramps begin and you should feel relief in minutes. Eating a banana morning and night is helpful, as well. Calcium tablets with magnesium and zinc also give good results.

## Low Energy

*Bananas* contain the natural sugars, sucrose, fructose and glucose along with fiber. A banana gives an instant and substantially-sustained boost of energy.

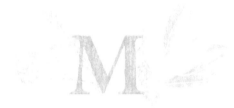

## Migraine Headache

Research shows high doses of riboflavin *(400 mg of Vitamin B-2)* can prevent migraines when compared to a placebo (*Neurology* magazine, Feb. 1998). *Feverfew* has been shown effective in treating migraines, 2 capsules 2 to 3 times per day. *Magnesium*, a mineral (300 mg once or twice daily) is also helpful for some migraine sufferers.

## Motion Sickness

Both *Ginger capsules* and *Candied Ginger* are very helpful. So is *Ginger tea,* made from fresh or dried ginger. However, ginger-flavored drinks such as ginger ale (which contains no ginger) don't work. Motion-sickness bands from the pharmacy are claimed to be effective, as well.

## Mouth Ulcers
(SEE ALSO HERPES)

A gargle made from *Snapdragon* (Antirrhinum majus): 2 cups Snapdragon flowers, or flowers and leaves, added to 4 cups boiling water and simmer for 5 minutes. Cool until a comfortable temperature, then gargle and spit out. Keep extra in the refrigerator for up to a week, repeating as needed.

## Nail Fungus

My formula, **Herbal Nail Fungus Soak**® is a reliable solution and it's guaranteed. Having a doctor remove your nails doesn't work - often if the nail grows back, which isn't unusual, the fungus comes back, too. Nail fungus often begins with an injury to the nail, like stubbing your toe on a rock. Fungus starts and is easily transferred to other nails by nail files or trimmers. Vicks Vaporub® works for some, although it's very slow (a year or more of daily applications). The best option - order **Herbal Nail Fungus Soak**® from LongCreekHerbs.com. It's guaranteed to work!

## Nasal Congestion
### (see also Coughing with Congestion)

**Fresh Ginger Root Tea** - Ginger helps open the nose and soothes the throat. Peel and slice a piece of fresh ginger root about the size of your thumb. Put the ginger slices in a pan with 4 cups water and simmer for 5 minutes. Let cool, strain. Sip a cup of the liquid, sweetened with honey if desired, 3 times daily.

**Apple Cider Vinegar & Garlic Tea** - Simmer 3 cups water, 2 cloves crushed garlic, 3 teaspoons dried oregano, 2 tablespoons apple cider vinegar and 1/2 teaspoon salt for about 3 minutes. Let cool, then sip 1 cup of this tea 3 times a day (also inhale the steam as you drink the liquid).

## Nausea

**Apple Cider vinegar or white wine vinegar**, 1 tablespoon in a 6 oz. glass of water. **Dill pickle juice** - Sip about 1/2 cup slowly - people swear by this!

Strong **Peppermint tea** (2 teaspoons peppermint leaves steeped in 1 cup boiling water for 10 minutes; don't add sugar or honey). **Peppermint oil** -Apply a drop to your finger and rub it on your gums. The fragrance is refreshing and helps ease nausea.

***Cinnamon-Rice water*** - Boil 1/2 cup (rinsed) rice in 2 1/2 cups of water for 10 minutes. Strain out rice and put aside for other use. To the rice water add 1 teaspoon cinnamon and drink 1/2 cup while still warm and another 1/2 cup every hour until you feel relief.

***Cinnamon-mint tea*** - Bring 2 cups of water to boiling, add 2 teaspoons peppermint or spearmint tea leaves and one 4-inch stick of cinnamon (or 1/2 teaspoon ground cinnamon). Remove from heat, cover with lid and let cool. Strain and drink 1/2 cup twice daily.

## NIGHTMARES, CHILDREN OR ADULTS

***No Nightmares Dream Blend*** - It may not sound logical but fragrance has been proven to have an effect on both mood and dreaming. My book, *Making Herbal Dream Pillows* gives details about dreams, both good dreams and nightmares. In the early 1980s I was given a no-nightmare dream blend from a practicing apothecary pharmacist, Jerry Stamps. Over the years I've recommended the formula to thousands of people and it works for nearly everyone. Here's the formula:

    1 tablespoon sweet hops
    1 tablespoon roses
    1 tablespoon lavender
    2 teaspoons marjoram

Mix together and place in a muslin drawstring bag (or even in a clean handkerchief, tied closed). Place this anywhere in the bottom of your pillowcase. The fragrance will be subtle but you'll find your nightmares will cease. To learn more about how Dream Pillows work, read my books: *Making Herbal Dream Pillows* (Storey Publishing), *Pillows & Potions,* and *Profits from Dream Pillows,* which are all available from LongCreekHerbs.com. Ready-made Dream Pillows are available there, too.

## NOSEBLEED

Sit straight up and tip your head slightly forward. Using your thumb and forefinger, firmly pinch the soft part of your nose shut and keep it there for a fully 10 minutes. Applying an ice pack can also help, (but not at the same time as pinching your nose). If it hasn't stopped by that time, see a doctor.

**Car Keys** - Dangle a set of car keys down the person's back. Lots of people swear by this. It probably works because the keys are somewhat cold, causing the person to cringe, which seems to help stop the nosebleed.

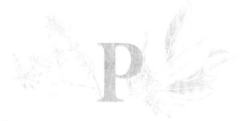

## Paper Cut

*Crazy Glue* or *Chap Stick*, applied to the cut.

## Pinkeye

Conjunctivitis, or pinkeye, is an inflammation of the inner eyelid and eye membrane and although it isn't generally serious, it is highly contagious. The Itching and swelling are unpleasant and should be seen by a doctor. While you wait for your appointment, try this. Fresh **Plantain** *(Plantago major)* leaves, bruised and applied as a poultice directly to the closed eyelids is helpful. A cool washcloth soaked in a solution of the herbs **Eyebright, Fennel seed or Chamomile**, also helps: Pour 1 cup boiling water over 2 teaspoons of dried Eyebright herb or 2 teaspoons dry Fennel seed. Cover and let cool for 20 minutes. Soak a wash cloth in the liquid and apply several times, 5 minutes each. This helps reduce the swelling and itching.

## Panic Attack

Here's a simple remedy that helps ease the feelings of panic. Put a drop of **German chamomile** *(Anthemis nobils)* essential oil in the palm of each hand. Rub your hands together then place them over your face. Begin slowly breathing and counting your exhaled breaths. German chamomile is known to be a calming fragrance. If that's not available, breathing into a paper bag slowly often helps. So does rubbing a bit of **Lavender essential oil** on the temples of each side of your head and inhaling the fragrance from your hands.

## PMS

Eat a *banana*! They contain Vitamin B-6 which regulates blood glucose levels and can affect mood and is often helpful. Two to three bananas a day is recommended. Also, this **PMS Symptom Relief formula** has proven helpful for some women: 1 cup Dandelion Root, 1 cup Burdock Root, 1/2 cup Chaste Tree berry (Vitex) and 1/8 cup dried Ginger. Mix and store in an air-tight container. To use: take out 1 heaping tablespoon of mix and simmer in 1 1/2 cups boiling water for 15 minutes. Drink 3-4 cups daily.

## Poison Ivy

When you come in contact with poison ivy, wash the exposed area immediately (within 10 minutes) with **dish soap and water**. Soap breaks up the oil that causes your skin to react. If you can't get to soap and water, cover the area with a damp washcloth until you can get somewhere with soap. Don't scratch - if you break the skin it will make the reaction worse.

**Jewel weed** *(Impatiens capensis)* is especially helpful in breaking up poison ivy oils that cause a reaction. Mash up the stems in your hands and rub the juice on the exposed area.

**Poison Ivy Wash** - Make sure of the identity of this herb before using it. It grows as a weed in lawns throughout most of the U.S. Pour 2 cups boiling water over 1/2 cup dried (or 1 cup fresh) **Plantain** *(Plantago major),* cover and let cool for 20 minutes. Strain out and discard the herb. Dip a clean wash cloth in the liquid and apply it to the affected area, repeating several times throughout the day.

## Psoriasis

There is supposedly no cure for psoriasis, but you can help avoid it or help your body recover more quickly and ease your symptoms with some simple home remedies. Drinking alcohol, being overweight, stress, a lingering case of strep throat, anxiety, some medicines, and sunburn all tend to make psoriasis worse. It's not contagious but for those who have it, it can be embarrassing and painful.

**Lemon Balm cream**, or decoction of lemon balm (see Herpes entry for directions) is often very helpful. **Cider vinegar** applied several times daily may help.

**Calendula oil** or Calendulated jel, from the pharmacy or whole foods store. **Zinc** ointment, that contains 10% zinc oxide, applied twice daily has shown to be helpful in reducing the redness and itching of psoriasis.

UVL treatments from a dermatologist are helpful but expensive; instead, lay in a *tanning bed* for 10-15 minutes. Or take **2000 IU Vitamin D3** supplements 4 times a day instead of the tanning bed.

This Skin Fungus formula holds some hope, as well: Mix 1/4 cup **Shavegrass**, 2 tablespoons **Lemon Balm**, 2 tablespoons **Lavender**, 1 tablespoon **Thyme** with 4 cups apple cider vinegar. Bring to a slow boil and let slowly simmer for 2-3 minutes. Remove from heat, cover with a lid and let cool overnight. Next day, strain and discard herbs and add 1 cup of plain water. Apply several times daily with washcloth.

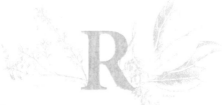

## Rashes, Diaper
### (Also see Skin Problems)

Most babies up to 24 months will have diaper rash at least once. Changing diapers more often helps. Strong detergents can also irritate, so change detergents, or use **vinegar** in the last rinse when washing cloth diapers. When rash develops, avoid disposable diaper-wipes, they contain alcohol which can make irritation worse and cause pain. Wash affected area with mild soap, rinse well and dry completely, then dust area with a powder that contains **zinc oxide**.

## Rashes, Adult

Adults, including those who are bed-ridden or incontinent, as well as healthy athletes, can develop a condition similar to diaper rash. Wash with as little soap as possible as it can further irritate, rinse well and let dry completely (use a hair dryer on low if necessary). Then apply this **Absorbent Powder** - Combine 1 cup cornstarch, 1 cup baking soda, 1 teaspoon zinc oxide (you can order it through the pharmacy or health food store), 25 drops Eucalyptus essential oil, 20 drops Mint essential oil and 12 drops White Thyme essential oil, in a zipper plastic bag and shake to mix. Apply to affected area 2 - 3 times a day to help with drying and healing. This is also an effective powder for itchy feet.

## Restless Leg Syndrome (RLS)

Putting a **bar of soap** under the bottom sheet of the bed is a method that thousands of people swear by. No one really knows why it works. The kind of soap used doesn't matter, any brand, wrapped or unwrapped. Place it underneath the bottom sheet in the area where your feet rest at night. It doesn't have to be under your feet, just nearby. Lots of people claim this worked like a miracle for them. Also eating a **banana** morning and night can be helpful.

## Ringworm

Ringworm or *tinea*, is an infection on the skin surface and looks like a reddish bumpy patch of skin; the center is white and appears to have a red "ring." It's a fungal infection, not a worm, and is caused by dermatophytes, which are parasitic fungi. These types of fungus survive on areas which are hot and moist. It's common, very contagious, and easily spread through direct contact with an infected person or pet. It can affect any part of the body. For example it's known as *tinea pedis* or "athlete's foot" on feet; on the groin is known as *tinea cruris* or "jock itch," on the body it's known as *tinea corporis*; and on the scalp, known as *tinea capitis*. If you have it in more than one area, which is common, you should treat all of the affected areas. You could apply over-the-counter antifungal lotions or creams that contain miconazole or clotrimazole, or make your own **Ringworm Treatment** - Combine 8 - 10 (peeled) raw Garlic cloves in a blender, with 1 tablespoon fresh Ginger root, 1 teaspoon Goldenseal root powder and 2 cups apple cider vinegar. Blend well and refrigerate.

Apply 3 - 4 times daily. Also drink 2 cups of Antifungal Tea, below, daily for 5 days.

***Antifungal Tea*** - This is helpful in the healing process, as well: Combine 2 teaspoons Lemongrass, 2 teaspoons Chamomile and 1 teaspoon fresh Ginger, with 3 cups boiling water. Simmer for 2 minutes, cover pan with lid and let cool for 10 minutes. Strain and drink 1/2 cup twice daily.

For athlete's foot and cracking heel, use my **Herbal Nail Fungus Soak**, available from LongCreekHerbs.com (it also works on jock itch, too). Most people see results in about 2 weeks.

**Tea Tree Oil** - Paint the oil on the affected skin areas 2 to 3 times daily, repeat until the ringworm is gone. Tea tree oil is considered non-toxic but some people may be allergic to it, so check a small area first.

One old time remedy I learned from the late Billy Joe Tatum, author of *Billy Joe Tatum's Wild Foods Field Guide and Cookbook*, was green walnut hulls. Mash up a green walnut hull and rub the juice on the ringworm-affected area. Repeat every day and in about 10 days the ringworm will disappear (although the stain from the green walnut hulls may last for a bit longer). ***Tobacco juice*** from chewing tobacco applied daily was my Granddad Long's remedy.

## SCALP, DANDRUFF AND SEBORRHEIC DERMATITIS

Seborrheic dermatitis and bad dandruff are caused by microscopic yeast fungi called Malassezia. There are medicated shampoos on the market that are effective. Just as effective, and less expensive, is ***apple cider vinegar***. Dilute it with equal parts water and pour over the hair after shampooing. Leave on the hair 7-10 minutes, then rinse. Apply every week and the condition should disappear in a few weeks. Continue applying once a month thereafter to prevent the fungus from returning.

This Skin Fungus formula is also helpful on face, skin or scalp: Mix 1/4 cup **Shavegrass**, 2 tablespoons **Lemon Balm**, 2 tablespoons **Lavender**, 1 tablespoon **Thyme** with 4 cups apple cider vinegar. Heat to a slow simmer and continue for 2-3 minutes. Remove from heat, cover with a lid and let cool overnight. Next day, strain and discard herbs and add 1 cup of plain water. For places on face or beard, apply several times daily with cotton ball or wash cloth. For hair, pour through, cover with a towel and leave on for 15 minutes. Don't rinse out.

## SCARS, PREVENTING

My pharmacist-cousin, Glenn Foster in Tennessee, recommends applying this lotion as soon as a wound has closed and is beginning to heal. It keeps the wound moisturized and helps prevent scarring. **Glenn's Scar Lotion** - In a small saucepan, slowly heat 2 teaspoons **Olive Oil** and 2 teaspoons **Wheat Germ Oil**. Add 2/3 ounce **Cocoa Butter** and heat, stirring, until melted. Pour the lotion into a container and allow to cool. Apply 2 - 3 times daily.

## SKIN PROBLEMS

**Calendula Salve** - Calendula has anti-inflammatory effects when used topically and also has antibacterial and antiviral qualities. For use on "problem skin" as well as rashes, diaper rash, chapped lips, cuts and scrapes, dry or itchy skin, make the following Calendula Salve - Combine 1/4 cup dry Calendula petals, 1/2 cup sunflower oil (or almond, avocado oils, etc.) and 1 tablespoon dried Lavender flowers, in the top of a double boiler. Simmer on very low for about 3 hours - you want the oil hot but not boiling. Strain the oil, squeeze out the flowers and discard them. Return oil to top of double boiler and add 1/8 cup grated beeswax. Slowly simmer until beeswax is dissolved. Pour into small containers and let cool. Your salve is now ready to use and will keep for about a year. Apply after every diaper change; rub a little on rashes or other skin problems. This is an excellent salve for small cuts and scrapes on kids or adults, and helpful on any kind of dry, patchy skin problems.

## Sleeplessness

**Valerian** is an herb that is gentle, safe and helpful in helping a person fall asleep. Usually 3-4 capsules thirty minutes before bedtime is recommended. (Valerian is also available as a "combination" formula that includes Valerian, Passionflower, Hops and Lemon Balm, and this works even better). **Chamomile tea** also helps one relax; drink a cup before bedtime.

**Dream pillows**, especially if the formula includes hops, is helpful for people who are restless or have nightmares and trouble sleeping. Hops is a mild sedative and safe to use with adults and children. (See also *Nightmares* for a source for Dream blends).

## Smelly Feet (or underarms and General Body Odor doesn't need to be in bold)

From *Ann Landers* newspaper column, many years ago: Zinc tablets, 2 daily for a week. Eating 2 bananas a day will accomplish the same thing; chlorophyll tablets, or Parsley Tincture, also help.

## Snoring

There are many dental devices, ranging in price from thirty dollars to over a thousand dollars. Many claim they help. Here are a few things that may also help:

1- If you're overweight, lose 10% of your body weight.

2- Avoid alcohol within 3 hours of bedtime.

3- Sleep on your left side, which keeps your tongue from blocking the airway.

## Sinus Infections

Daphne Miller, MD, a physician in San Francisco and author of *The Jungle Effect: A Doctor Discovers the Healthiest Diets from Around the World* suggests that many sinus infections can be treated with a simple saline nasal wash instead of antibiotics. She suggests dissolving **1/4 teaspoon plain table salt and 1/4 teaspoon baking soda** in a cup of purified lukewarm water. Inhale a bit of the solution about one inch up into your nose, one nostril at a time by sniffing the solution out of the palm of your hand. Then very gently blow your nose, being careful not to hurt your ears. Repeat the process with the other nostril and continue alternating nostrils until your nose is clear. Do this rinse twice daily until the condition improves.

## Sore Gums

*Thyme* is an effective remedy for sore gums. It has antiseptic properties and is used as a germ-killer in mouthwashes. Use the following mouthwash to help heal mouth irritations and relieve sore, inflamed gums. (Swollen gums are often an indication of infection, so don't put off seeing a dentist, but meanwhile, this is an excellent remedy with no known side effects or cautions).

**Thyme Mouth Rinse** - Gather 1 cup fresh Thyme leaves and stems, or use 1/2 cup dried Thyme leaves. Bring 4 cups of water to boil. Add the Thyme, stir, and remove the pan from heat. Cover the pan with a lid and let cool overnight. The following day, strain out and discard the Thyme, saving the liquid. Add 1/3 cup cheap vodka to prevent the mixture from fermenting or going sour (or use 1 cup pasteurized apple cider vinegar instead). This can be kept in the refrigerator for a month or more.

**To use:** After brushing your teeth, morning and evening, take about an ounce (a shot glass full) in your mouth and swish it around for about 30 seconds then spit out. You should see improvement in 2-3 days. Keep using the mouthwash a couple of times a week to prevent the infection from returning. This also sweetens bad breath!

## Sore Muscles

1/4 cup dry **Ginger** (or 1/2 cup chopped fresh) added to a warm bath. Ginger has anti-inflammatory properties that help aching muscles heal. Soak for 10 minutes to help relieve the soreness. Repeat once daily until soreness is gone.

According to Chris Black, PhD, Professor of Kinesiology at Georgia College and State University, who has been studying ginger for relieving muscle soreness, "You could use ginger any place or time you'd normally take a pain-relieving medication...the amount of pain reduction using ginger is comparable, if not better, than similar studies that use ibuprofen, aspirin or naproxen." Taking **2 teaspoons of dried or fresh ginger** as a tea or in a beverage before and after working out, is as effective as over-the-counter pain relievers. Also, drink plenty of fluids. Muscles get sore from lactic acid buildup, according to David Govaker, M.D., Corporate Medical Director for Humana in Louisville, Ky. Staying hydrated will help wash the lactic acid out of aching muscles.

## Sore Throat (also see Coughing)

Sore throat is often caused by an infection. The American Dental Association suggests you replace your toothbrush every 3 months, and especially replace it after a sore throat to avoid reinfection. Soak your toothbrush in a solution of 2 teaspoons plain bleach in 1/3 cup of water for 5 minutes to help kill any germs.

Also helpful is this **Ginger Mouthwash** - Combine 2 level tablespoons freshly-grated ginger, 1 tablespoon fresh lime or lemon juice and 2 teaspoons honey with 2 cups boiling water. Cover pan and let cool for 10 minutes. Leave ginger in, it will settle to the bottom. Sip on this hot mixture throughout the day.

## Spider Bite (Brown Recluse)

According to Tina Marie Wilcox, head gardener and herbalist at the Ozark Folk Center State Park in Mountain View, AR, this **Oatmeal poultice** is helpful: Add a heaping 1/2 cup old-fashioned oats to 1 cup of boiling water and cook for 3 minutes. Remove pan from heat and add 2 tablespoons **Goldenseal root** powder, 6 large finely chopped fresh **Comfrey leaves** and 1 tablespoon of **Echinacea tincture** and mix. Apply it as soon as the spider bite is discovered. She changes the poultice (held on with a cloth bandage) 2 or 3 times a day. She recommends monitoring body temperature and general physical condition and to seek medical advice immediately if first aid is not proving effective.

## Sprains

**Snapdragon Compress** *(Antirrhinum majus)* - Boil 3 cups of fresh snapdragon flowers and leaves in 8 cups water. Simmer slowly for 15 minutes. Strain (or leave in) the herbs. Apply the liquid as a very warm compress, (or washcloth) leaving on for 15 minutes. Repeat 3 times a day.

## STRESS & DIFFICULTY SLEEPING

*Lemon Balm tea* (Melissa officinalis), a lemony scented herb with a long history of easing anxiety, helping with memory and aiding in sleep. According to Eric Yarnell, ND, an assistant professor of botanical medicine at Bastyr University in Kenmore, WA, "Lemon Balm appears to calm an overactive thyroid, also known as Graves' disease. The herb also speeds healing of oral herpes lesions." For tea, put 2 teaspoons dried Lemon Balm in a cup and pour 1 cup of boiling water over. Cover and let steep for 5 minutes, strain and drink about 30 minutes before bedtime. *Also see listings under* **Nightmares** *and* **Sleeplessness**.

## SUNBURN

*Aloe Vera*, fresh from the plant or bottled, applied liberally several times a day. Dr. Thomas Westbrook Lynch, MD PC, a dermatologist in Springfield, MO, recommends ***an aspirin*** dissolved in 1/2 cup water and applied to the skin as an emergency treatment.

***Snapdragon Balm***: 1 cup chopped Snapdragon flowers and leaves, 1 cup chopped Plantain leaves *(Plantago major)* in the top of a double boiler with 3 cups of sunflower, avocado or almond oil. Let slowly simmer (but not boil) over low very heat for 30 minutes. Cover and let sit overnight. The following day, strain out and discard herbs. Add 2 teaspoons Vitamin E oil. Apply as needed. ***Raw cucumber***, rubbed on the skin is also soothing.

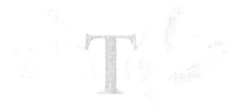

## TOOTHACHE

A toothache is an indication of a problem with the tooth and you need to see a dentist. However if you have to wait several days for an appointment, this old-time remedy can help. Suck on a ***whole clove***. Or apply a drop of clove oil (also called Eugenol) with a cotton bud. Clove oil has antiseptic properties which can help fight infection, and also has a numbing effect.

## Upset Stomach

**Fennel tea** is effective; so is **Peppermint** or **Spearmint tea**. A few drops of **Marshmallow** *(Althaea officinalis)* tincture in a fourth cup of water is also effective. Herbal tinctures containing those herbs are available from health foods stores.

## Urinary Tract Infection (UTI)

**Baking Soda** - To prevent UTI or stop it at the first symptom, drink 1 teaspoon baking soda in a glass of water 2 or 3 times daily. The soda neutralizes the acidity in your urine, helping with recovery.

**Blueberries** - Eat them often on your cereal. Blueberries and cranberries are from the same plant family genus *Vaccinium*. Drinking blueberry or 3 - 6 ounces of ***cranberry juice*** daily is a good preventative for UTIs.

**Parsley** - As far back as 1629, folk healers recommended *Parsley* for urinary tract infections. In 2002 it was reported beneficial in the *World Journal of Urology*, in a review of animal studies using Parsley roots for increasing urine output. The *German Commission E* has approved Parsley root for cystitis and related urinary tract problems: Drink daily cups of tea made from 2 tablespoons common Parsley (root and/or leaves). Pour 2 cups of boiling water over and let steep for 5 minutes, strain and drink. You can also find Parsley tincture at health foods stores. To help with the healing, add chopped Parsley leaves to salads and soups.

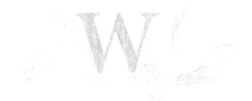

## Warts

Wash effected area in plain *apple cider vinegar*. Let dry without rinsing then apply *duct tape* to warts and leave the tape on. Do this daily and in a few weeks the warts should be gone.

*Banana peel*, applied white side next to the skin and held in place with tape has also proven effective. When the peel turns black, replace it with another until the wart is gone.

Terry Willard, a medical herbalist, claims his favorite remedy is the fresh, white juice from *Dandelion* stems. Pick a dandelion stem, split it open and apply it to the wart. Repeat 2 - 3 times a day for 7 to 10 days.

The inside of the leaf of Hens & Chicks (Sempervivum sp) is said to work well, too. Apply and hold in place with tape.

## Weak Fingernails/Toenails

Soak your nails in a small container of *olive oil* for a 4-5 minutes each day. Massage the oil well into the cuticles, then pat dry, and drink 3 cups daily of *Nettles and Oatstraw Tea* - 2 tablespoons each: dried Nettles and Oat straw over which you pour 1 cup of boiling water. Cover and let steep for 15 minutes, strain and drink.

*Fingernail Hardener* - Mix 3 tablespoons water, 1 tablespoon glycerine mixed with 1 teaspoon powdered alum and store in an airtight container. **To use:** before going to bed, using a small brush, apply some to each nail and let dry. The following morning, remove with rubbing alcohol and apply hand lotion to hands and nails. Repeat for several nights or as needed.

## Worrying, Constant

If you're stuck in a constant worry mode it can prevent you from making useful decisions. Try this: Put 3 or 4 drops of *Sandalwood essential oil* on your chest. Close your eyes and sitting up straight in a chair with your hands in your lap, breathe slowly and count as your breathing goes in and out. Keep this up for about 10 minutes or until you feel your tension begin to ease. Instead of sandalwood, a few drops of lavender oil applied to your temples and hands, can also be relaxing.

## Wrinkles

Blend one *ripe banana* in a cup of milk and drink twice daily to help with skin problems. In addition to that, mash 1/4 *banana* into a paste. Smooth it on the face and leave for 15 minutes. Rinse with warm water, then splash on cold water. Do this once a week to tighten skin.

Combine 1 envelope *Knox Unflavored Gelatin* with a little warm water to make a paste. Smooth it on the face and let dry. After 10 minutes, wash it off and your skin will feel much tighter.

## Yeast Infection, Vaginal

Yeast infections can appear anywhere on the body including between the toes, underarms, fingernails, etc. The most common form is vaginal yeast infection. Try this: Combine 2 cups water, 1 tablespoon apple cider vinegar and 2 cloves of freshly-crushed Garlic cloves. Leave overnight, strain out garlic and apply as a douche.

This treatment is also very effective: Fungus Fighter (Spilanthes-Usnea Tincture), available from LongCreekHerbs.com.

# Resources

*American Journal of Clinical Nutrition*

*An Honest Herbal* by Dr. Verro Tyler

*Body Care Just for Men*, Jim Long

*Digestive Wellness*, by Liz Lipski, PhD

*Making Herbal Dream Pillows*, Storey Pub.; Jim Long

New York University Medical Center (med.nyu.edu)

*Neurology* magazine

*Prevention* magazine

*The Green Pharmacy* by Dr. James Duke

*The Jungle Effect: A Doctor Discovers the Healthiest Diets from Around the World*, Dr. Daphne Miller, MD

The People's Pharmacy

Rodale.com

WebMD

Zorba Pastor on Your Health (wpr.org/zorba)

# INDEX

Acid Indigestion ................. 1
Acid Reflux ..................... 1
Arthritis........................ 2
Bad Breath...................... 2
Bed Bugs ....................... 3
Bed Sores ...................... 3
Bee Sting ...................... 3
Bitten Tongue ................... 4
Bleeding........................ 4
Blood Pressure .................. 4
Body Odor....................... 4
Boils ........................... 5
Brittle Nails .................... 5
Bruises ......................... 6
Burns .......................... 6
Burnt Tongue ................... 6
Burn from Eating Hot Pepper ..... 7
Canker Sores.................... 7
Chigger Bite..................... 7
Constipation .................... 7
Coughing........................ 8
Coughing, Dry ................... 9
Coughing with a Cold/Congestion .. 9
Coughing, Nighttime.............. 9
Cracking Heel.................... 9
Cuts & Scrapes .................. 10
Dandruff ....................... 10
Depression...................... 11
Diarrhea........................ 11
Diaper Rash (see Rashes) ........ 12
Earache......................... 12
Erectile Dysfunction ............ 12
Eyes, Puffy...................... 12
Flatulence, Gas ................. 13
Fleas on Pets or People .......... 13
Gout ........................... 13
Hair Conditioning ............... 14
Hair, Split Ends, Damaged Hair ... 15
Hangover....................... 15
Heartburn ...................... 15
Hemorrhoids.................... 15
Hemorrhoids, External, Internal ... 16
Herpes, Genital or Oral........... 16
Hiccups ........................ 16
Insect Bites..................... 17
Itching Eyes (also see Pinkeye) .... 17
Irritable Bowel Syndrome ........ 17
Jock Itch........................ 18
Leg Cramps..................... 18
Low Energy..................... 19
Migraine Headache .............. 19
Motion Sickness................. 19
Mouth Ulcers (see also Herpes).... 19
Nail Fungus..................... 20
Nasal Congestion (see also
Coughing with Congestion) ....... 20
Nausea ......................... 20
Nightmares ..................... 21
Nosebleed ...................... 21
Paper Cut....................... 22
Pinkeye......................... 22
Panic Attack .................... 22
PMS ........................... 23
Poison Ivy ...................... 23
Psoriasis........................ 23
Rashes, Diaper .................. 24
Rashes, Adult ................... 25
Restless Leg Syndrome........... 25
Ringworm ...................... 25
Scalp, Dandruff, Seborrheic
Dermatitis......................26
Scars, preventing................ 27
Skin Problems................... 27
Sleeplessness ................... 28
Smelly Feet ..................... 28
Snoring......................... 28
Sinus Infections ................. 28
Sore Gums...................... 29
Sore Muscles ................... 29
Sore Throat .................... 30
Spider Bite...................... 30
Sprains ......................... 30
Stress & Difficulty Sleeping....... 31
Sunburn........................ 31
Toothache ..................... 31
Upset Stomach ................. 32
Urinary Tract Infection .......... 32
Warts .......................... 33
Weak Fingernails/Toenails ....... 33
Worrying, Constant.............. 33
Wrinkles........................ 34
Yeast Infection, Vaginal.......... 34
Resources....................... 35

# Notes

Scan this QR code at the left with a smartphone to view the author's video showing how his Herbal Nail Fungus Soak® is used.

## More books from Jim Long:

Best Dressed Salads

Dream Pillows & Potions

Easy Dips Using Herbs

Easy Homemade Crackers Using Herbs

Fabulous Herb & Flower Sorbets

Great Herb Mixes You Can Make

Growing & Using the Top 10 Most Popular Herbs

Handy Guide to Nail Fungus

Herbal Cosmetics

Herbal Medicines of the Civil War

Herbal Medicines of the Santa Fe Trail

Herbs, Just for Fun

How to Eat a Rose

It Will Do No Harm to Try It,
the Home Remedies Diary of Elias Slagle

Make Your Own Hot Sauce

Make Your Own Romantic Bentwood Trellises

Making Herbal Vinegars

Profits from Dream Pillows

Recipes & Food from the Civil War

Sensational Salsas from Apple to Zucchini

Books available through distributors, in herb and gift shops and from his website: LongCreekHerbs.com; wholesale information for businesses upon request.